Dedicated to my sons, Christopher and Ethan, and all the children of the world to inspire and nurture their knowledge of their gifts within and that of the world they live in.

Note to readers. We have written this book to appeal to children of all ages. Older children can try the yoga poses and activities on their own, but we suggest that parents help and supervise younger children. It is much more fun if two or more children do the activities together.

First published by Our Street Books, 2014
Our Street Books is an imprint of John Hunt Publishing Ltd.,Laurel House, Station Approach,
Alresford, Hants, SO24 9JH, UK
office1@jhpbooks.net
www.johnhuntpublishing.com
www.ourstreet-books.com

For distributor details and how to order please visit the 'Ordering' section on our website.

Text copyright: Dawattie Basdeo 2014

ISBN: 978 1 78279 819 4

A CIP catalogue record for this book is available from the British Library.

Illustrations and design: Angela Cutler

Printed and bound by CPI Group (UK) Ltd, Croydon, CR0 4YY

We operate a distinctive and ethical publishing philosophy in all areas of our business, from our global network of authors to production
and worldwide distribution.

For further information on Holistic World™ and Holistic World Yoga Kids visit www.holisticworld.co.uk
To see more of the illustrator's work, visit souls-heart.blogspot.co.uk

Public Liability Disclaimer
The author nor the publisher cannot accept responsibility for, or shall be liable for, any accident, injury, loss or damage, including any
consequential loss that results from using the ideas, information, procedures or advice offered in this book.

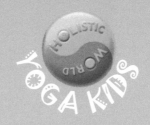

Natural World Treasures Young Yogi Series

Magnificent Me, Magnificent You
The Grand Canyon

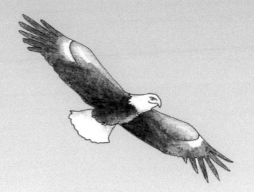

Written by Dawattie Basdeo
Illustrated by Angela Cutler

OUR STREET
BOOKS

Winchester, UK
Washington, USA

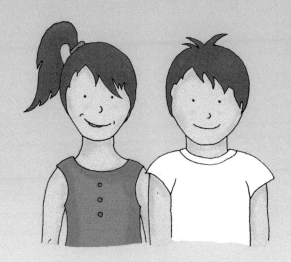

Meet twins Crystal and Leo.

They invite you on their journey...

Salute to the Sun

The sun salutation (Surya Nama) is a wonderful, flowing sequence of yoga postures to warm up, wake up and energise all the muscles of your body.

1. Stand in the **mountain pose**, your feet together and your hands at your sides, feel tall and strong like a mountain. Breathe in and bring your palms together at the centre of your heart into the **prayer position**. As you stand, feel the ground solid beneath your feet and take a few deep breaths in and out as you calm and focus your mind.

2. Breathing in, raise your arms above your head and reach for the sky. Look up to the sky through your open arms.

3. Breathing out, flow your arms down in a circle around your body resting on the outside of each foot with your fingers pointing forwards in line with the toes of your feet. If needed you can bend your knees slightly. Let your head hang towards the floor like a rag doll.

4. On an in breath, step your **left foot** back into a lunge.

5. On an out breath, step your **right foot** back to join your left foot into the **plank position**. Your body should be in a straight line with your arms straight below your shoulders and toes pointing forward.

6. On an out breath, lower to the **staff pose**. Lower your body to floor with your elbows bent and your chin gently touching the ground.

7. On an in breath, push gently forwards into **cobra pose**. Look up and straighten your elbows by pushing against the floor. Raise your chest up and draw back your shoulders. Take a few deep breaths.

8. On an out breath, tuck your toes under to point forwards, and push up through your arms lifting your hips up to the sky into **downward dog pose**. Take a few deep breaths in this position whilst pushing down equally between your feet and your arms.

9. On an in breath, step your **right foot** forwards between your hands into a lunge position.

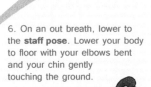
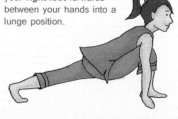
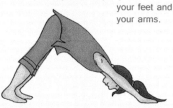
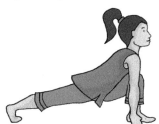
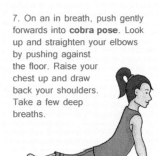

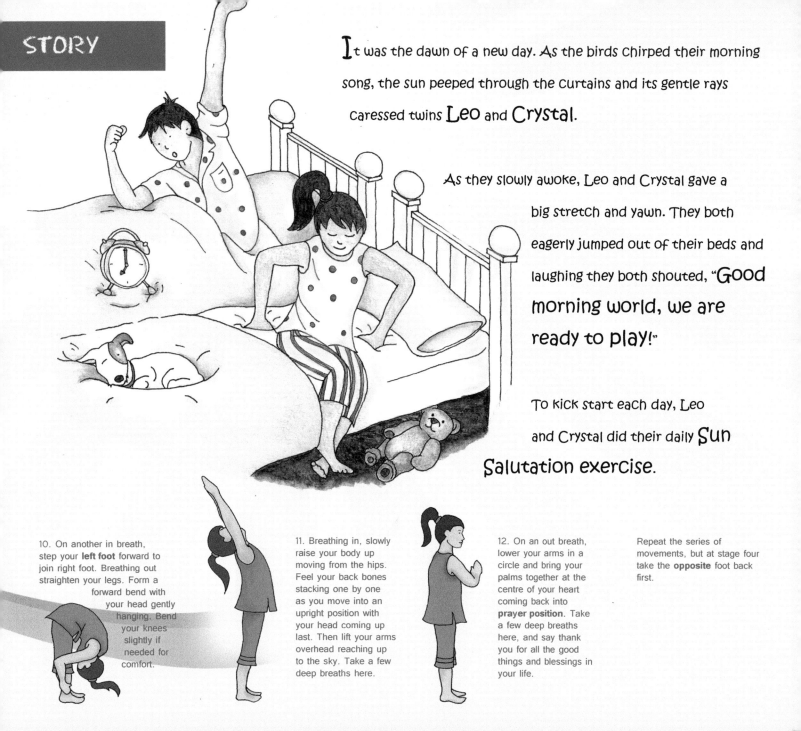

It was the dawn of a new day. As the birds chirped their morning song, the sun peeped through the curtains and its gentle rays caressed twins Leo and Crystal.

As they slowly awoke, Leo and Crystal gave a big stretch and yawn. They both eagerly jumped out of their beds and laughing they both shouted, "Good morning world, we are ready to play!"

To kick start each day, Leo and Crystal did their daily Sun Salutation exercise.

10. On another in breath, step your **left foot** forward to join right foot. Breathing out straighten your legs. Form a forward bend with your head gently hanging. Bend your knees slightly if needed for comfort.

11. Breathing in, slowly raise your body up moving from the hips. Feel your back bones stacking one by one as you move into an upright position with your head coming up last. Then lift your arms overhead reaching up to the sky. Take a few deep breaths here.

12. On an out breath, lower your arms in a circle and bring your palms together at the centre of your heart coming back into **prayer position**. Take a few deep breaths here, and say thank you for all the good things and blessings in your life.

Repeat the series of movements, but at stage four take the **opposite** foot back first.

"What shall we do today?" said Leo.

"Let's visit somewhere from Mummy's bag of travelling treasures."

"Great idea!" said Leo, "Let me choose something."

Crystal held the bag while Leo excitedly rummaged inside with his hands.

Slowly he pulled out a treasure and held it up.

"What's that?" asked Crystal.

"It's a feather!" said Leo.

They both looked at the feather. It was long and smooth and the plume was a warm brown colour with a reddish golden patch and white squares on the tip.

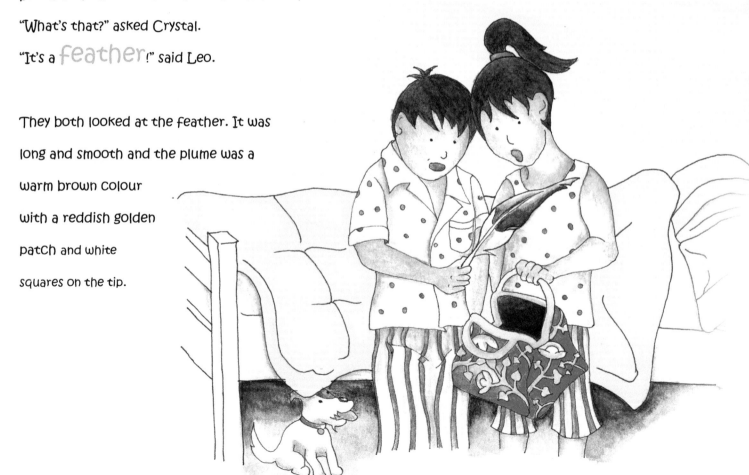

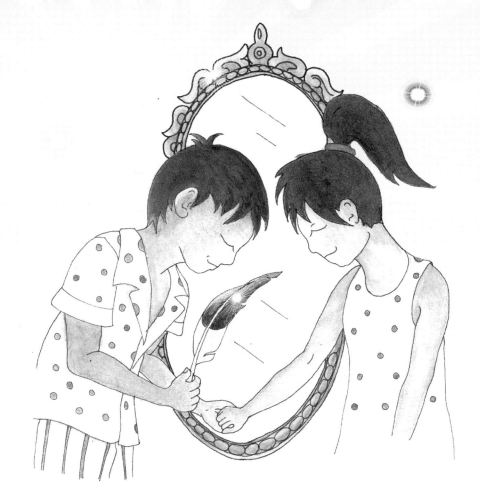

"Let's use our wishing mirror to find out who it belongs to."

Quickly they ran over to their wishing mirror, stood in front of

it, closed their eyes, wished and said, "Mirror, mirror, take us to

the **owner** of this feather."

Feather Breathing Meditation

Breathing is an essential activity to keep us alive! In yoga, we learn to become aware of how we breathe so that we can connect our mind and body.

Sit tall in an upright position with a straight back, but sit comfortably. This is called the 'easy pose'. The hands are placed gently resting on each knee, or with the first finger and thumb touching which is called 'chin mudra'. A mudra is a hand position in yoga which means 'lock' or 'seal'. In yogic science each area of the hand relates to a certain area of the brain. In applying pressure to the fingers and hands, the related brain areas are stimulated. The chin mudra corresponds to the area that activates wisdom and knowledge.

As you sit in the 'easy pose', focus on your breathing. Take a few deep breaths in and out to calm and focus your mind.

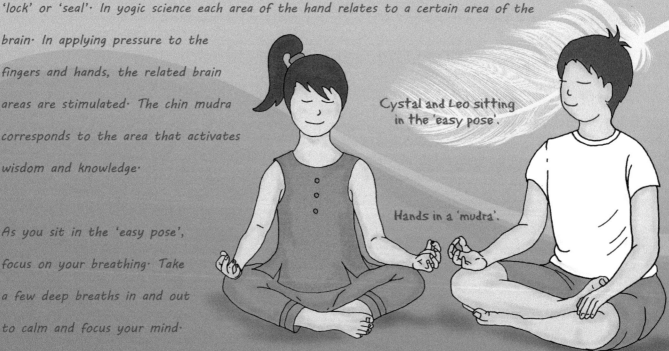

Breath in deeply

Breath out slowly

Cystal and Leo sitting in the 'easy pose'.

Hands in a 'mudra'.

Breathe in deeply through your nose and out slowly through your nose. Now, imagine what it feels like to be a feather…soft, light, gentle, calm, peaceful and floaty. When calm and focussed start the breathing exercise below.

To begin, breathe in, take a deep breath for a count of three or five, whichever feels comfortable. As you breathe in, feel your stomach expand with your breath. In your mind say, 'Breathing in, I relax all the muscles in my body'.

When filled with breath, hold it for a count of two or four which ever feels comfortable. Then gently breathe out for a count of three or five whichever you find most comfortable. Whilst breathing out, say in your mind, 'I feel full of peace and light like a feather'.

Repeat this breathing exercise five times.

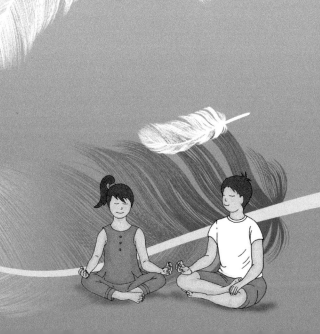

When they opened their eyes, they found they were standing in the middle of a **Native American village**. The village was a bustle of activity, full of tipi's, children playing, men grooming their horses and women cooking.

As they looked around they spotted an old man playing with his dog. He wore a headdress made of similar feathers to the one they held. They quickly went over to him, greeting him with their hands in prayer position. They bowed and asked him if he could help them find the owner of their feather.

The man was one of the wise elders of the village. He wore a warm kind smile. and his sun kissed face was covered with wisdom wrinkles.

He said, "The owner of this feather is truly magnificent and very sacred to my tribe, I know where you can find what you seek. But before you set off on your journey, let us join with the some of the warriors of my tribe and do our **Eagle Dance** to wish you wisdom and strength for your journey."

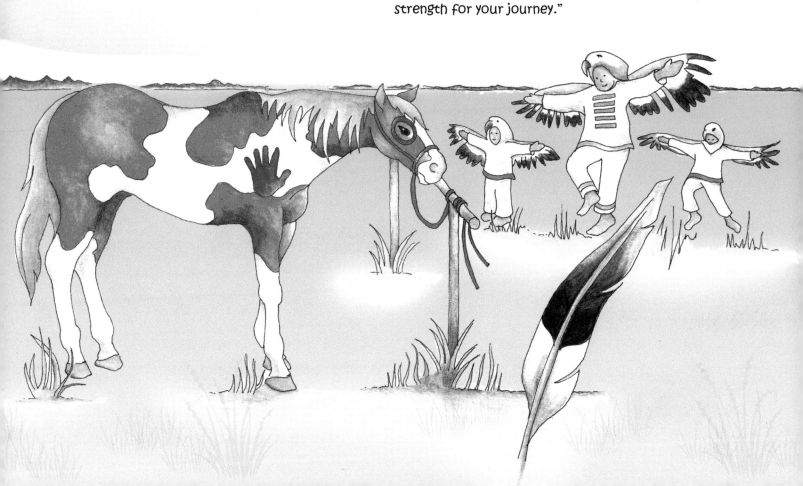

Native American Eagle Dance

Native Americans use dance for many purposes and it is an important part of their lives. It is used as a way to pray, express grief or joy, seek connection with nature and spirits, honour everything from birth to marriage to death, heal sickness, prepare for war and to tell stories.

This is our version of the Native American Eagle Dance. You can make your own costumes to pretend to be an eagle.

Dance sticks can be used. Original dance sticks were usually made of wood with a section of antler on one or both ends of the stick, with feathers symbolising prayers sent to the 'Great Spirit'.

Some members of the group can sit to the side and be musicians and singers. You can use drums and shakers or tambourines to beat a steady rhythm.

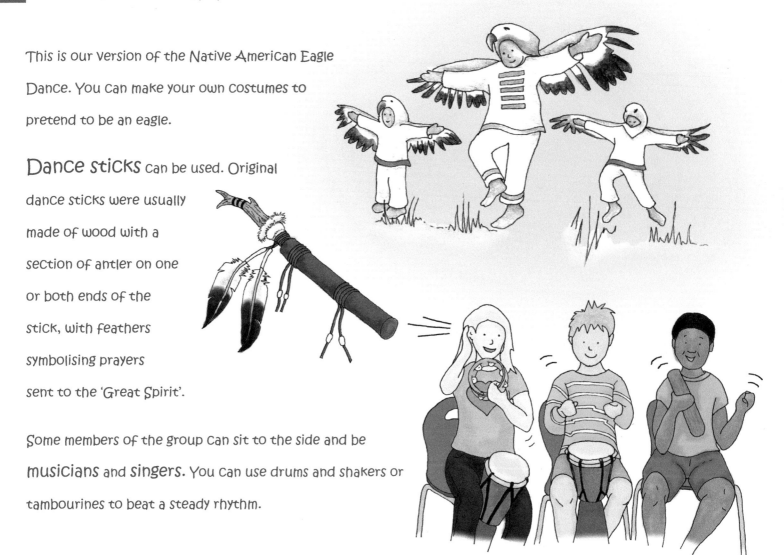

IMAGINE. Before you begin the dance, imagine what it must be like to be an **eagle in flight**, and use your imagination to think of dance moves based around the movements of the eagle.

The dancers form a circle. Two dancers stand in the centre of the circle and perform imitations of eagle movements.

The remaining dancers form a circle around them, and start dancing to their own imagined beat or to the rhythm of the music, moving in a clockwise direction.

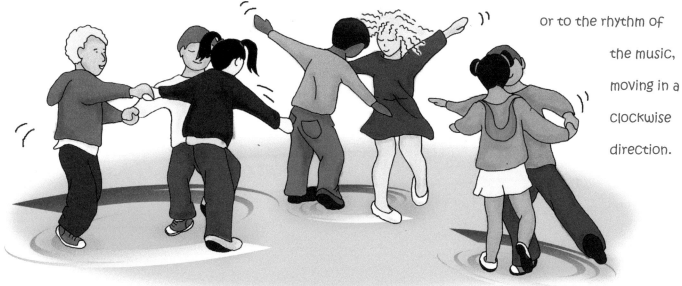

Some suggested dance moves are flapping wings, spinning around in a circle, letting out eagle cries, hopping from one foot to the other, shuffling along and bobbing up and down to the beat. **Freely express yourself** through whichever movements come to your imagination. At intervals change direction from clockwise to anticlockwise and back again.

And most of all, let go and have fun!

Warrior II Pose

The warrior pose (Virabhadrasana II) is a dynamic yoga stance that provides energy and strength for both the mind and body. It helps tone and strengthens your thighs, shoulders, back, neck and stomach muscles.

Pretend to be a brave Indian warrior.

1. Stand in the **mountain pose**, breathing in and out. Feel strong and grounded like a mountain.

2a. Breathing in, jump or step your feet apart sideways. Hold your body upright. Take a few breaths and feel strong, proud and confident in yourself.

2b. Breathing in, raise your arms sideways until they are in line with your shoulders, palms facing down. Keep your shoulders relaxed. Feel the stretch across both of your arms.

3. Keep your **left foot** facing forwards and **swivel your right foot** towards the right. On an out breath, lower your body slightly. Keeping your back leg straight and strong, bend your right leg into a **lunge pose** with your knee positioned above your ankle, forming a right angle with your leg.

4. Next, turn your neck and your face towards the direction of your front foot. Take a few deep breaths in this position and gaze ahead in the direction of your fingers. Become aware of how strong your legs and torso feel. Holding this pose, feel powerful and focussed in your mind.

5. On an out breath lower your arms, straighten your legs back to the **astride pose** (picture 2). With your toes pointing forwards, gently jump or walk feet back together into the **mountain pose**.

In order to balance out our body, repeat the exercise, this time turning your other foot forwards and facing in the opposite direction.

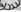

Crystal and Leo felt exhilarated and **strong like warriors** after doing the **Eagle Dance**.

As they thanked the villagers and set off on their journey, the wise old man said, "Yes, the owner of this feather is truly magnificent, but **within you** there is also a **treasure trove of magnificence**, that will support you to achieve your heart's desire.

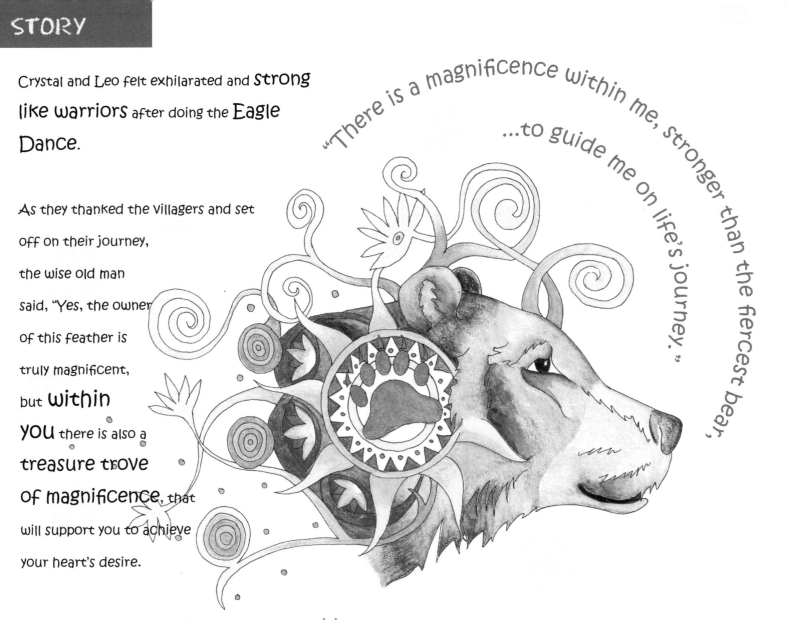

"There is a magnificence within me, stronger than the fiercest bear, ...to guide me on life's journey."

If you feel afraid on your journey, here is a positive mantra you can say to yourself to remind you of your **power within**."

The first part of their journey began with them travelling down a river with the assistance of a kind villager in his canoe. Sitting in the canoe as it gently glided over the flowing clear water, they both felt a sense of peace and calm.

Crystal looked at the water below, admiring the sparkles made by the sun bouncing of it and the rainbow coloured fishes swimming in it. "The water is beautiful," she said in awe.

"Yes," said the canoe man, "it remains beautiful because it is in constant flow, thus avoiding the water becoming sluggish, murky and polluted. It is the same with life. Change supports the cycle of life. As we are unable to grasp water in our hands, so we are unable to grasp and stop life's flow. Change is part of life, we have to go with life's flow and know it is all for the greater good."

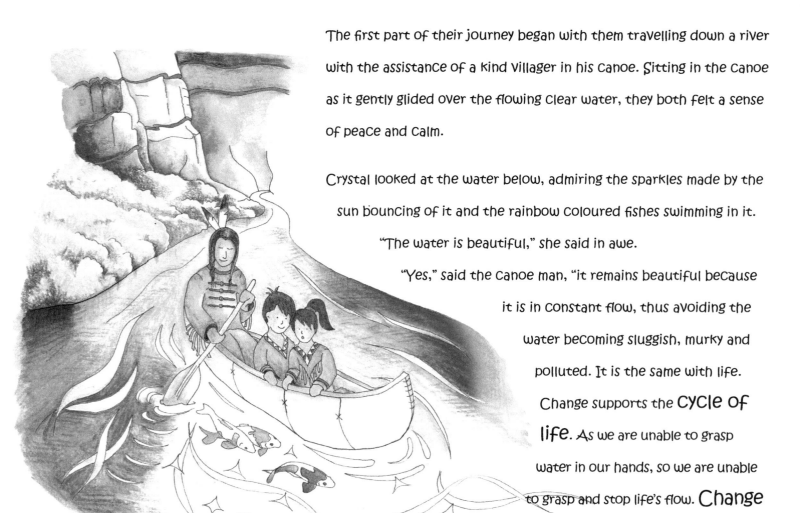

As they thought about what the canoe man said, a song came to Leo, and he shared it with his companions. They all sang it as they continued to the end of their journey by canoe, where they thanked and waved goodbye to the kind and wise canoe man.

Boat Pose

The boat pose (Navasana) is strong dynamic yoga pose that will build up the strength of your stomach muscles.

Imagine you are a sailing boat powering through the waves.

1. Sit on the floor with your legs straight in front of you and your torso upright. Press your hands to the floor a little behind your hips with your fingers pointing towards your feet. Sit tall and lean back. Take a few breaths here as you find your point of balance.

3. Keeping your arms straight, stretch your arms out parallel to the floor, holding them on the outside of your legs with your fingers pointing forwards.

Take a few in and out breaths holding the pose for a few seconds as long as you are comfortable to do so.

2. On an out breath, bend your knees and lift your feet off the floor. Point your legs and feet upwards towards the sky at an angle that feels comfortable for you.

4. On an out breath, lower your legs to the floor, and breathing in, sit back upright being aware of the strength in your body.

Leo's Song

This is the song

Leo created, which they all sang

together as they were rowed

down the river.

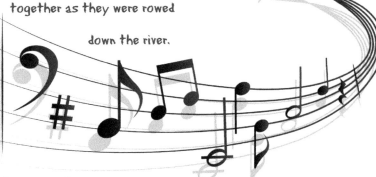

Can you make up a

lilting, flowing tune to go along with the words?

If there is a group of children, form a circle holding hands, sway and bob about, imagine you are in a boat riding the crest of the waves as you all sing. During the chorus, use your arms to send a wave flow around the circle. You can reverse the direction of flow for the second chorus.

You can still do these activities if you are on your own.

River of Life Song

We're on the River of Life
We're on the River of Life
The waves go up, the waves go down
On the river of life
The river of life

There is no controlling it
You have just got to roll with it
Just go with the flow
Knowing it's the Cycle of Life
Don't You Know

Chorus

We are on the River of Life
We are on the River of Life
The waves go up, the waves go down
On the river of life
The river of life

Sometimes the waters get rough
And life just seems a bit tough
Just keep rolling, just keep flowing
Knowing it's the cycle of life
The cycle of life

Repeat chorus

Sometimes the waters gently flow
And your heart is set aglow
Just keep rolling, just keep flowing
Knowing it's the cycle of life
The cycle of life

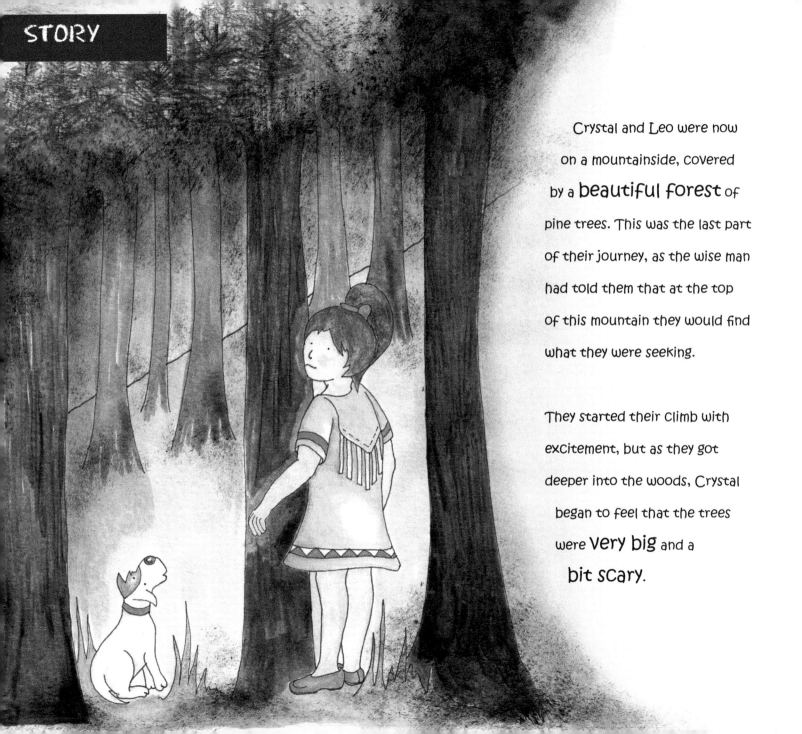

Crystal and Leo were now on a mountainside, covered by a **beautiful forest** of pine trees. This was the last part of their journey, as the wise man had told them that at the top of this mountain they would find what they were seeking.

They started their climb with excitement, but as they got deeper into the woods, Crystal began to feel that the trees were **very big** and a **bit scary.**

Leo laughed, "You do not have to be afraid of trees – they are our friends.

Trees are the lungs of our planet, they produce the oxygen that we breathe to stay alive."

"Wow!" said Crystal, and she ran to a tree giving it a hug and said, "Thank you, trees, thank you, plants."

And she felt a sense of wonder and humbleness under the canopy of beautiful pine trees.

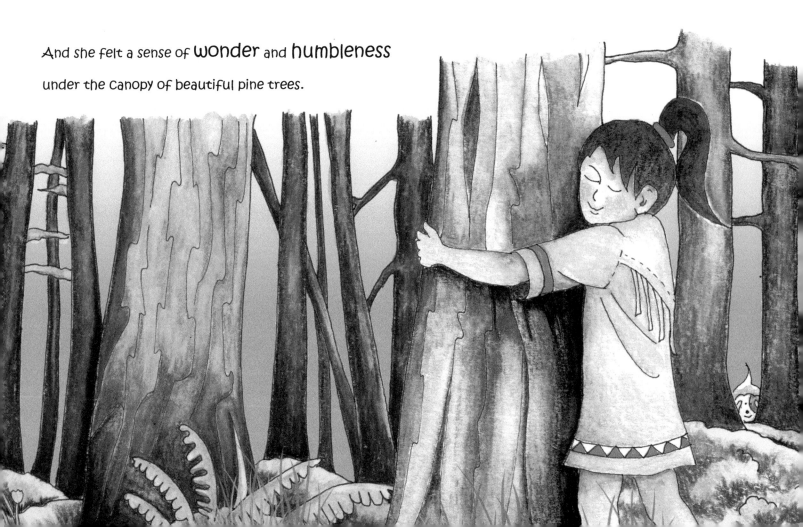

Tree Pose

The tree yoga pose (Vriksasana) helps to bring balance and clarity to the mind, and strengthens legs and ankles.

Feel your feet rooted into the earth and your arms reaching up like branches.

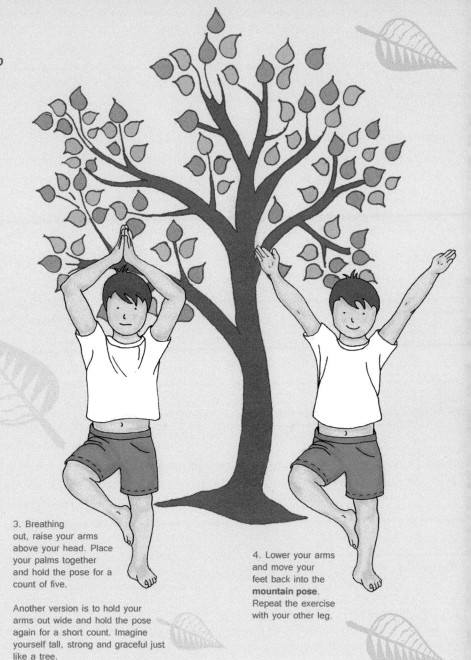

1. Stand in the **mountain pose**, keep your body and head upright. Imagine being strong and solid like a mountain. Breathing in, bring your hands into **prayer position** holding them at the centre of your heart. Feel peaceful and calm.

2. Breathing in, place your **right foot** on the inside of your left leg wherever feels comfortable, but not against your knee.

3. Breathing out, raise your arms above your head. Place your palms together and hold the pose for a count of five.

Another version is to hold your arms out wide and hold the pose again for a short count. Imagine yourself tall, strong and graceful just like a tree.

4. Lower your arms and move your feet back into the **mountain pose**. Repeat the exercise with your other leg.

Bear in the Woods Game

A game to have fun, create laughter and practice yoga poses.

One child pretends to be the bear and placing themselves in the middle of the room, curled up like a sleeping bear. The other children in the group stand at one end of the room and have to tip-toe over to the other side of the room past the sleeping bear.

The bear can wake up every now and then and then go back to sleep. Each time the group of children think the bear is stirring to wake up, they have to pretend to be a tree and stand in the tree pose. If the bear sees any child that is not in tree pose, that child gets turned to stone and has to assume rock pose.

Tree pose

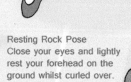

Resting Rock Pose
Close your eyes and lightly rest your forehead on the ground whilst curled over.

Once all the children have crossed to opposite end of room the game can be repeated with another child as the bear.

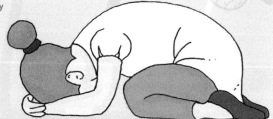

Curl up and pretend to be a sleeping bear

Suddenly through the trees, they both spotted a sleeping black bear.

They both felt a little afraid, but they remembered

the mantra the wise man of the village had told them to say

when they were afraid.

They **repeated** this in their **minds** as they

slowly crept past the bear. Anytime the bear

appeared to stir, they stood still and quiet just like a

tree until they had gone well past him.

"There is a magnificence within me, stronger than the fiercest bear, ...to guide me on life's journey."

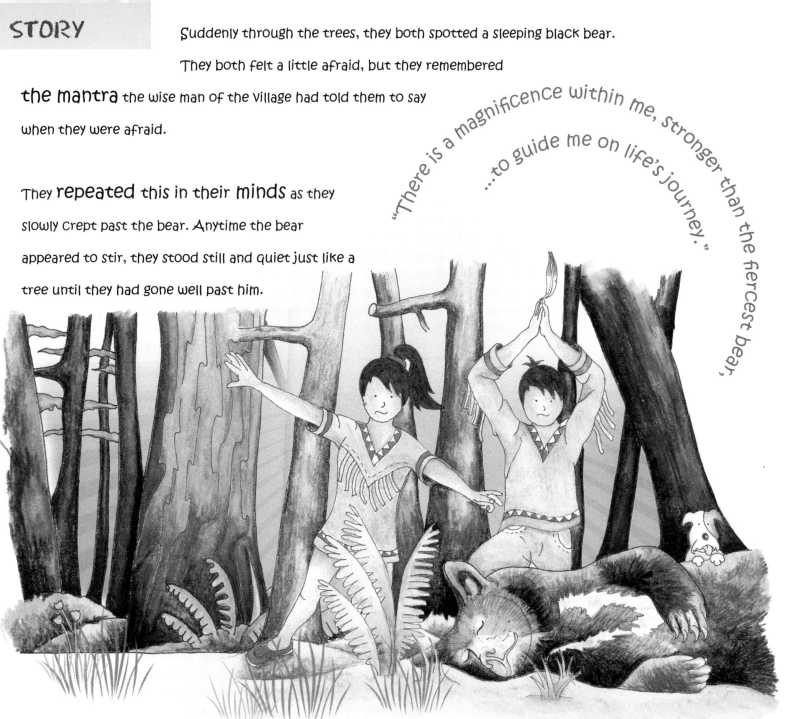

At last they reached the top of the mountain. As they stood at the top, taking in a deep breath, they surveyed their surroundings.

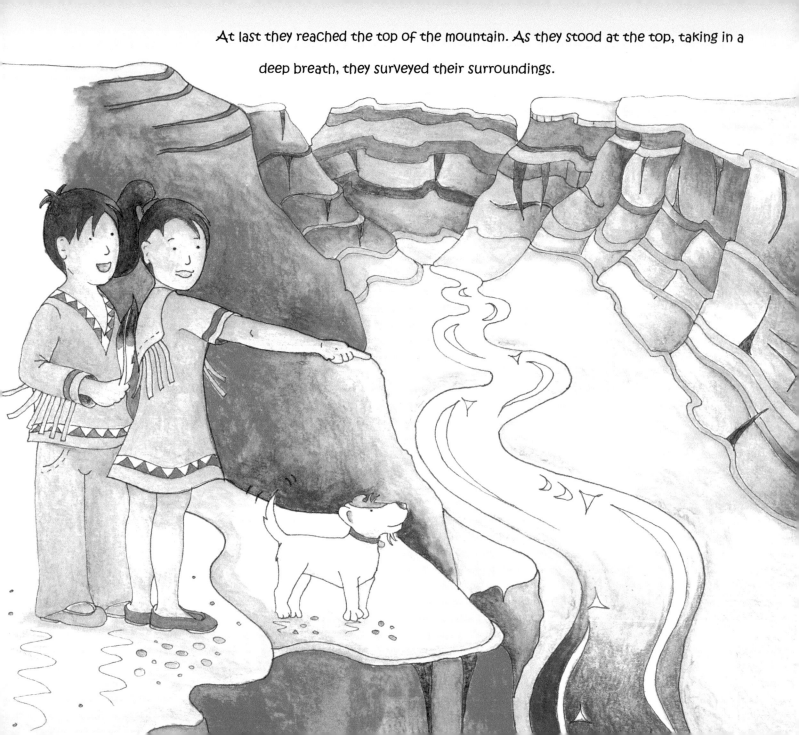

"**WOW!**" they said in unison, as they looked down and around at the spectacular **magnificence** of the Grand Canyon. "It's **amazing**," said Crystal, "that water, so pure, flowing and fluid has carved all these hard mountains into these spectacular shapes through time.

"Yes," said Leo, "it goes to show that we can achieve great things in time. We must **believe** in our **abilities** and **FOCUS** on our **goals**. Then by taking continuous action, in time, we will be able to **carve out our dreams.**"

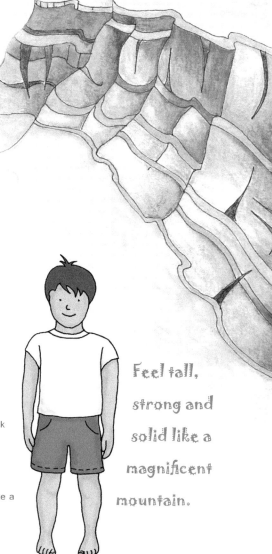

ACTIVITY

Mountain Pose

Mountain yoga pose (Tadasana) helps to improve posture, strengthens legs, back and stomach muscles.

1. Stand tall and proud with your head upright and your shoulders back.

2. Spread your toes and allow them to feel **firmly connected to the ground**. Sway gently back, forth and sideways and then stand still, be aware of feeling balanced and grounded.

3. Breathing in, become aware of the strength in your thigh muscles.

4. Breathing out, pull your shoulders back and open your chest area. Allow your arms to hang by your side.

5. As you hold this posture breath in and out deeply a few times. **Imagine youself feeling tall, strong and solid** like a **magnificent mountain**.

Feel tall, strong and solid like a magnificent mountain.

Eagle Pose

Eagle yoga pose (Garudasana) improves your balance and strengthens your shoulders and thighs.

1. Stand in **mountain pose**.

2. Breathing in, raise your arms in front of you up to shoulder level with palms facing up.

3. Cross your left arm over your right arm. Bend your arms at the elbow and wrap your forearms around each other, bringing your palms together with fingers pointing up towards the sky.

4. Breathing out, slightly bend your knees and shift your body weight to your left leg.

5. Breathing in, cross your right leg over your left thigh, and hook your right foot around your left calf.

6. Hold this position and take a few slow in and out breaths. Feel yourself calm, balanced and focussed like an eagle.

7. Breathing out, release your arms and legs back into the **mountain pose**.

8. Repeat this pose using your opposite arms and legs in order to balance your body.

Feel balanced and focussed like an eagle.

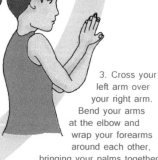
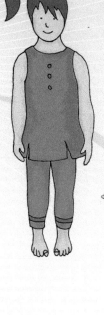
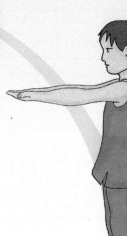

Then from up above they heard a chirping whistle,

"Kleek kik it ikik". They looked up and there,

soaring above them in splendid glory was the bald eagle, the magnificent

owner of the feather.

Crystal held up the feather to the wind and waved it at the eagle.

The feather, although soft and delicate, belonged to a

bird of true magnificent strength and agility.

As the bald

eagle with his white

crown on his head soared and

swooped, Leo and Crystal felt a warm

sense of happiness and gratitude to have

found the owner of their feather treasure.

They held hands, closed their eyes, and took a deep breath of

the fresh mountain air. A feeling of bliss filled them both.

When they opened their eyes, they were back in their bedroom.

Leo and Crystal excitedly ran to their mum to tell her of their adventure.

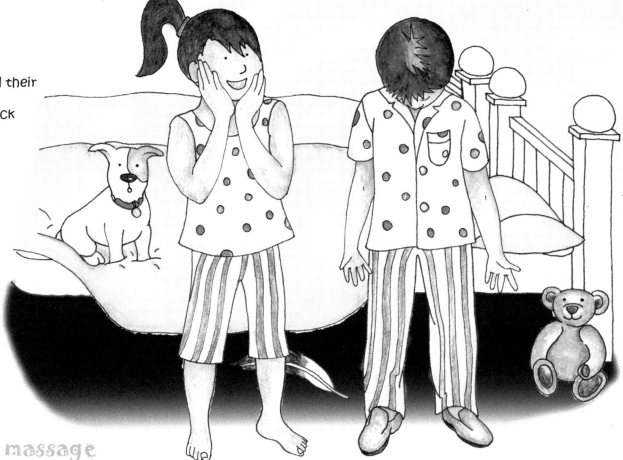

Back massage

Before you start ask your partner if it is okay to massage them. Massage is a wonderful relaxing way to connect with your friend. Here are several different ideas for massage play. Always make sure movements are gentle.

1. Sunrise – Make big circular movements on your friend's back using the palms of your hands. This warms up the back, just like the sun warms us.

2. Feather – Spread your fingers and place them in the centre of your friend's back on either side of the spine and make a pulling motion out towards their sides, as if stroking along a feather's quill. Repeat these movements up and down back.

They shared their adventure by playing it out on her back giving her a gentle massage.

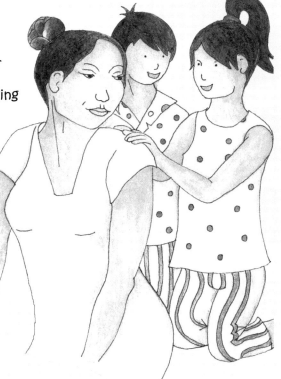

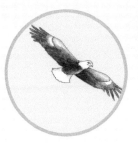

7. Flying Eagle – Use your fingertips to make gentle flying taps around your friend's back.

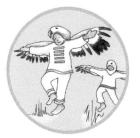

3. Native American Villagers Eagle Dance – Dance your fingertips around your friend's back, moving your hands in a circle clockwise and then anticlockwise direction.

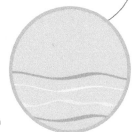

5. River – Use the sides of your hands to make wave like movements on your friend's back.

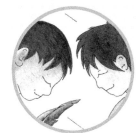

8. Closing Eyes and Returning Home – Gently stroke down your friend's back with your fingers.

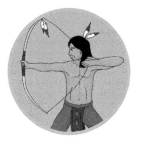

4. Warrior – Make gentle chopping movements on your friend's back using the sides of your hands.

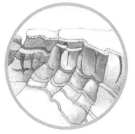

6.Climbing Mountain – Use your knuckles or fingertips to walk up your friend's back.

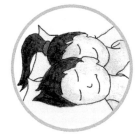

9. Sleep – Rest your palms for a few seconds at the bottom of your friend's back to end the massage.

Flight of an Eagle Guided Meditation

Sit comfortably in easy pose.

Close your eyes and breathe gently in and out through your nose.

Allow your body to feel relaxed, but keep your mind alert.

Now imagine you are standing at the top of a Grand Canyon mountain.

Imagine you are looking out at the vastness surrounding you.

As you breathe in, you can feel the warmth of the sun

on your body.

It rejuvenates and invigorates all the

cells of your body.

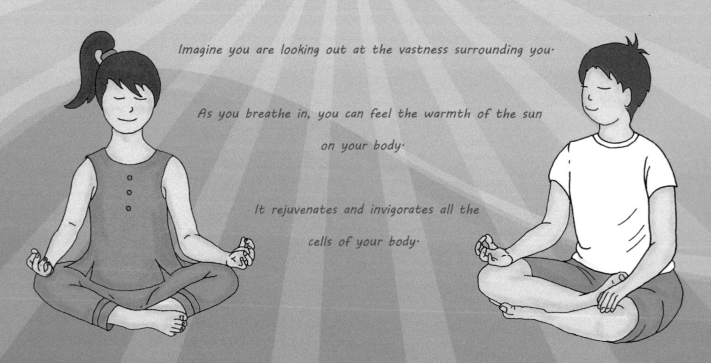

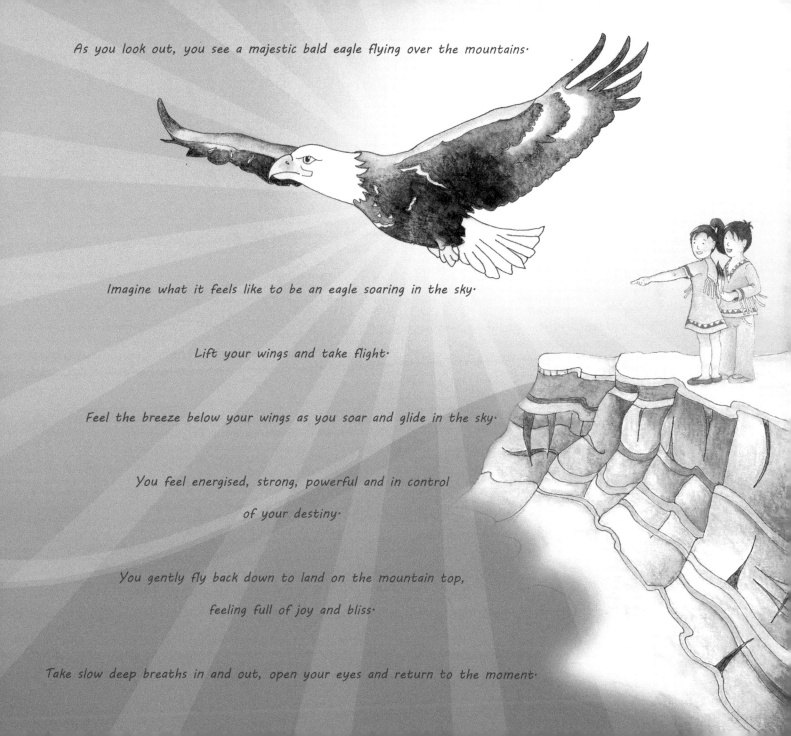

As you look out, you see a majestic bald eagle flying over the mountains.

Imagine what it feels like to be an eagle soaring in the sky.

Lift your wings and take flight.

Feel the breeze below your wings as you soar and glide in the sky.

You feel energised, strong, powerful and in control
of your destiny.

You gently fly back down to land on the mountain top,
feeling full of joy and bliss.

Take slow deep breaths in and out, open your eyes and return to the moment.

When they were finished recounting their day's adventure their mum tucked them into their warm cosy beds. Before they fell asleep they said their Native American peace poem:

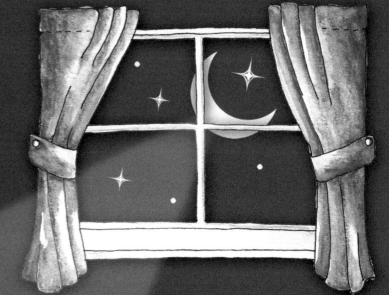

Let us know peace

For as long as the moon shall rise

Let us know peace

For as long as the rivers shall flow

Let us know peace

For as long as the sun shall shine

Let us know peace

For as long as the grass shall grow

Let us know peace.

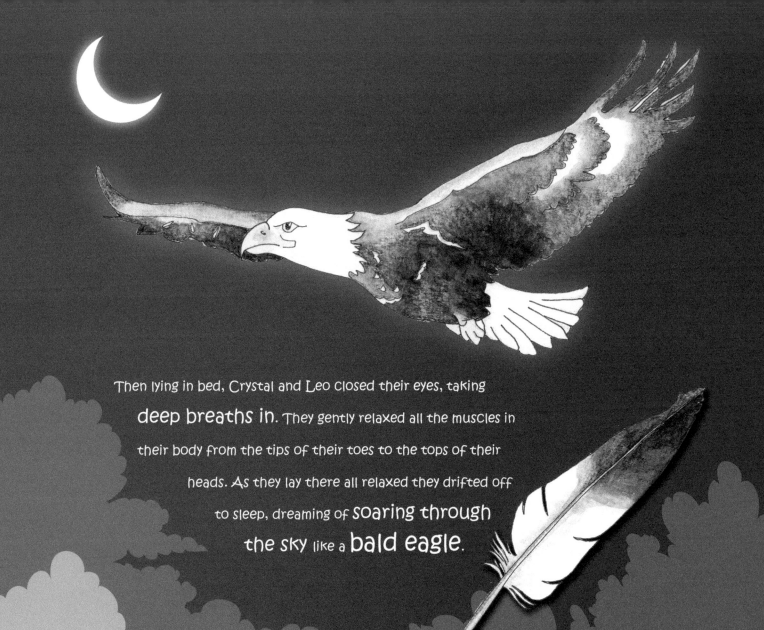

Then lying in bed, Crystal and Leo closed their eyes, taking **deep breaths in.** They gently relaxed all the muscles in their body from the tips of their toes to the tops of their heads. As they lay there all relaxed they drifted off to sleep, dreaming of **soaring through the sky** like a **bald eagle.**

Interesting fast facts page

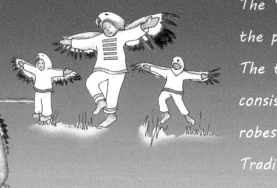

The Grand Canyon is 277 miles (446km) long.

Evidence suggests the Colorado River established its course through the canyon at least 17 million years ago and continues to erode and form the canyon even today.

The Pinyon pine forests, with their distinctive fragrance, grow on both rims of the Canyon and Pinyon nuts were once a staple diet of the Native Americans.

Native American Indians have inhabited the area continuously for thousands of years.

The 'Hualapai tribe' translates to the people of 'Ponderosa pine.'

The traditional dress of Hualapai consists of deerskin and rabbit skin robes.

Traditional houses of the Hualapai are conical in shape, formed from cedar boughs called a Wikiup.

The Pueblo people considered the Grand Canyon a holy site and made pilgrimages to it.

The bald eagle derives its name from an old English word, 'balde', meaning 'white', as in 'white headed eagle'.

The bald eagle is the National bird of the U·S·A·

The bald eagle is a sacred bird in some North American cultures,
and its feathers are central to many religious and spiritual customs
among Native Americans·

Eagles are considered spiritual messengers between God and humans by some cultures·

The Bakota Native American tribe gives an eagle feather as a symbol of honour to a person who
achieves a task·

The Choctaw Native American tribe sees the bald eagle is a symbol of peace·

Many Native Americans represent the eagle in many of their dance moves·

Black bear is
one of the
many animals
inhabiting
the North
American
Colorado
area·

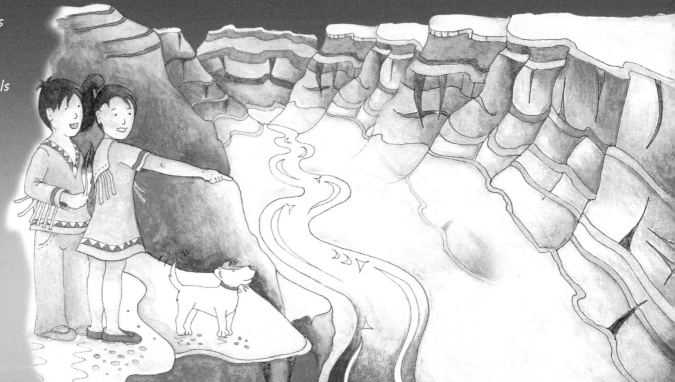

Where in the world?
Is the Grand Canyon?

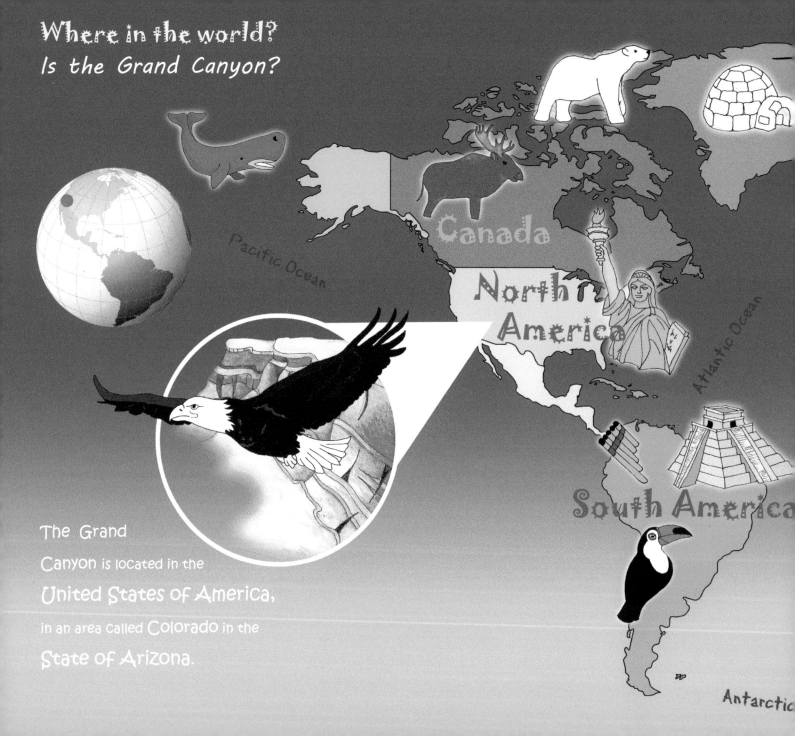

Canada

North America

Pacific Ocean

Atlantic Ocean

South America

Antarctica

The Grand
Canyon is located in the
United States of America,
in an area called Colorado in the
State of Arizona.

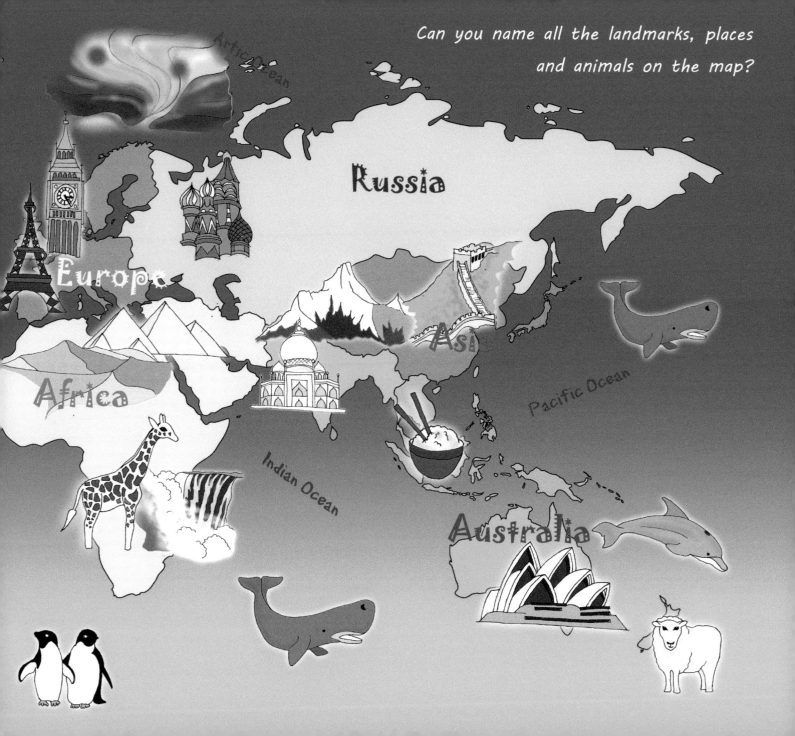

Can you name all the landmarks, places and animals on the map?

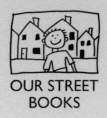

OUR STREET
BOOKS

Our Street Books for children of all ages, deliver a potent mix of

fantastic, rip-roaring adventure and fantasy stories to excite the

imagination; spiritual fiction to help the mind and the heart

grow; humorous stories to make the funny bone grow; historical

tales to evolve interest; and all manner of subjects that stretch

imagination, grab attention, inform, inspire and keep the pages

turning. Our subjects include Non-fiction and Fiction, Fantasy

and Science Fiction, Religious, Spiritual, Historical, Adventure,

Social Issues, Humour, Folk Tales and more.